RIDDLE OF HEART ATTACK & SEX:

THE ROLE OF SEX IN CARDIAC ARREST

JOHN D. GEISER

1

Table of content

INTRODUCTION

INTRODUCTION

Death, without a doubt, is a spirit, but it mostly relies on human bodily derangements to bring about the most dreadful catastrophe in human history. Surprisingly, heart attack has remained a "weapon of mass devastation" throughout its history. Millions of individuals have perished as a result of these well-studied and acknowledged health problems. Thousands of individuals are dying every day as a consequence of their ignorance about the same condition. If these conditions are avoidable or controllable, then follows that death is likewise preventable or may be postponed.

Chapter 1

THE MYSTERY OF HEART ATTACK

Heart Attack is responsible for most sudden mortality. It shows frequently; abrupt collapse and death after heavy exercise in a healthy-looking man or woman. Heart Attack is not a respecter of race or gender. On September 21, 1998 Americans were astonished when the fastest woman sprinter of all time, Florence Griffith Joyner, heretofore healthy seeming, died unexpectedly at the age of 38 of a heart attack.

What is Heart Attack?

Think of the heart as a Pumping Machine that pumps blood via a network of pipes (the blood veins) to supply oxygen to diverse tissues, including the heart muscle itself. The arteries that give blood to the heart itself are called **coronary arteries**. If there is damage or constriction (atherosclerosis) of the heart arteries over a while, it is called **coronary artery disease** or simply "**heart disease**". On the other hand, if there is sudden obstruction of the heart artery, the oxygen supply to the injured portion of the heart muscle may be partly or fully cut off. The latter which may lead to sudden death is called a heart attack. The latter ailment is technically called **Myocardial infarction**.

What Causes Heart Attack?

Most heart attacks are induced by a blockage in coronary arteries. Usually, the blockage is caused by **atherosclerosis**, which is the growth of fatty deposits (called plaque) inside the artery. This buildup is like the sludge that builds up in a drain pipe and slows the flow of water.

Heart attacks may also be induced by a blood clot that gets stuck in a tiny segment of an artery to the heart. Clots are more prone to form when atherosclerosis has left an artery narrow. It may also be caused by sudden spasm(contraction) of the coronary artery. The spasm may be brought on by stress, cold, or exertion. Also, Carbon monoxide from generator fumes may generate a situation of hypoxia (loss of oxygen) to the tissues which might injure the heart muscles leading to Heart Attack.

How Common Is Heart Attack?

Millions of people die yearly as a result of heart attack however its speedy start and insufficient post-mortem analysis have left most Africans guessing and occasionally choosing ignorantly on the probable explanation of the premature demise.

However, Statistics from the American Heart Association offers a heart-breaking study on America and heart attack. The poll indicates that every 20 seconds, someone in the US has a heart attack. Fortunately, because of great medical breakthroughs in recent decades, heart attacks are decreasingly fatal. Nonetheless, heart attack accounts for one-third of all deaths in women and it is also the top cause of mortality among Women over age 50 in America.

Angina Pectoris;

This is a mild heart attack characterized by reversible chest pain which may last up to five minutes. It also occurs with a sense of pressure or an impression of numbness or heaviness beneath the breastbone or across the chest.

It is largely caused by insufficient circulation and limited Oxygen supply to the heart muscles. It occurs in both males and women but is more frequent in women. It is alleviated by rest or by specialized treatment.

Chapter 2

RISK FACTORS FOR HEART ATTACK:

A heart attack does not simply occur. Certain disorders may leave the heart susceptible to assault. Those conditions are termed **risk factors**. There are around nine significant risk factors. All except age and family history are adjustable. Major risk factors for heart attack include;

Age:

The risk of heart attack and heart disorders grows directly with age. It happens more commonly in adults older than 45 years. Male inclination exists in adults aged 40-70 years. In adults older than 70 years, no sex predisposition occurs. In general, women begin suffering heart attacks 10 years later than males owing to the protective effects of the female hormone, estrogen, before menopause. However, following menopause, when the level of estrogen is low, the risk of heart attack rises. It is vital to realize that heart attack does not merely occur just because one is aged. No! Other predisposing variables play a major part.

Family History:

Heart attack runs in families; that is if you have a first-degree relative or parents who had a heart attack. This is primarily because disorders like Hypertension, and diabetes that stimulate the development of unhealthy circulatory systems also run in families.

Smoking:

There is no need to stress this matter. To an American Heart Association study; smoking triples the risk of a heart attack. Cigarette smoking also decreases the age for first heart attack more in women than in males. The Summary is that heart attack is the number one killer of Americans and most of the fatalities are smokers. It is based on the devastating consequences of Cigarette smoking on the heart that the World Health Organization created the phrase; *Cigarette Smokers are liable to die young.*

High Blood Pressure, Diabetes, and Obesity.

It is vital to highlight that hypertension, diabetes, and obesity drive approximately 90% of all fatalities that happened due to heart attacks. Elimination or management of this nuclear illness family preserves the heart in a healthy condition, all things being equal.

Elevated Cholesterol:

Cholesterol is s just small fat molecules. Fat taken into the body is utilized by the cells for energy in the form of cholesterol. There are two kinds of cholesterol; **LDL**, low-density lipoprotein, and **HDL**, High-Density Lipoprotein.

The former (LDL) is named bad cholesterol because it may induce blockage of blood vessels (arteriosclerosis) whereas HDL İs considered healthy cholesterol since it carries excess cholesterol from the cells and blood vessels to the liver for processing.

In overweight or obese persons, the cholesterol level is also high, hence the cause for the increased incidence of heart attack within the population. Interestingly, the amount of cholesterol may be determined by simple laboratory tests and addressed, if need be.

Lack of Exercise:

Physical inactivity increases a twofold risk of a heart attack. Studies reveal that regular exercise may cut the risk of heart attack by 40%. Mild to moderate exercise has been discovered to promote blood circulation, strengthen the heart, prevent blood clotting, aid regulate blood sugar, and also boost the 'good' Cholesterol (HDL).

Stress:

Stress and especially suppressed anger have been reported to raise blood pressure and heart rate. Stress puts increased stress on the heart and in the presence of other risk factors renders the heart prone to abrupt attack.

Race:

Heart attack has been observed to be higher among African Americans. This may not be linked with unguarded feeding habits and residual African mindset amongst the blacks.

Motherhood:

Due to inactivity associated with mothers after birth.

Depression:

While heart disorders or have had heart attacks may undoubtedly cause or contribute to depression, depression itself is a risk factor that can aggravate heart disease. Depression raises the chance of blood clot development (thrombus), which might cause a heart attack.

Vitamin Deficiency:

Certain vitamins have been discovered to be advantageous to the heart via their capacity to reduce a potentially detrimental chemical **"homocysteine'"** in the blood. Long-term data gathered on 80,000 women in America over a 14 year period indicated that women who drink at least 400 mg of folic acid per day and more than 3 mg of vitamin B6 may lower their risk of heart attack by about half. Also, low levels of vitamin B12 have been connected with increased **homocysteine** (harmful material) levels.

Vitamin E, an antioxidant, has been demonstrated to lower cardiac risk. Data is emerging indicating having appropriate calcium intake (1.500mg/day) for menopausal and postmenopausal Women is critical for good heart health as well as bone health. The wonderful thing here is that one may receive the daily Vitamins needed with correctly prepared daily multivitamins.

Infections:

Infections, notably, sore throat and skin infections, should be quickly treated since such infections may move to the heart and cause cardiac infections such as endocarditis or pericarditis which may induce a heart attack.

Chapter 3

SIGNS OF HEART ATTACK AND THEIR PREVENTION:

Just like any other sickness, a heart attack has indicators via which it might be detected. The traditional symptoms/signs of heart attack are;

- Crushing Chest Pain, *which may spread to the shoulder, to the jaw, or down the arm;*
- Shortness of Breath;
- Sweating;
- Nausea and or Vomiting;
- Dizziness;
- Rapid or Irregular Heartbeat
- Weakness.

Classically, these symptoms are generally brought on by physical activity or abrupt mental stress. Another major observation in heart attack is that the incidence of its occurrence rises between 4 am and 10 am. This is due to the release of the body's adrenaline during this period. In the US, This warning says; **if you experience chest discomfort with one or more of these symptoms go to the emergency hospital immediately.**

Although chest pain remains the most significant presenting Symptom, it is still vital to clarify that not every chest pain is a heart attack. No! There are several disorders, unrelated to the heart that might give rise to chest discomfort. few of these disorders are;

Anxiety	gallbladder	infection	heartburn
pneumonia	pleurisy	indigestion	peptic ulcer, etc.

From my tropical clinical experience, chest discomfort related to gastric ulcer, pleurisy, and indigestion are more prevalent. However, your doctor should make a correct diagnosis in this respect.

Prevention of Heart Attack

A heart attack is a serious emergency. It comprises a strong communication system, good ambulance facilities, a decent road, and good cardio-resuscitation facilities. Therefore, "Prevention" should continue to be the motto for the majority of Africans. The good news is that if certain precautions are taken, heart attacks may be avoided or at least reduced. This involves avoiding or reducing the risk factors.

Stop smoking.

This is the single most crucial factor in heart attack prevention. The manufacturers of tobacco are sweating because of laws that are against them everywhere except in Africa. The World Health Organization has done all possible to safeguard people against this risk, but since every person has the freedom to choose their path in life, they do not intervene.

The good news is that quitting smoking may reduce a person's risk of mortality from heart disease by 24% in only two years. Within three to five years of stopping, former smokers may begin to approach the risk level of a non-smoker.

Control your weight, blood pressure, and blood sugar

It is necessary to control these three heart attack relatives. They have been discussed extensively. If you are in control of these factors, you need not worry since a heart attack seldom happens without a risk factor.

Workout Your Body

It is important to note that light to moderate exercise encourages healthy blood circulation, inhibits blood clotting, and has additional advantages that lessen the impact of other Heart Attack risk factors.

Eat a nutritious diet.

Reduce your intake of foods high in sodium (salt) and saturated fat to decrease cholesterol and blood pressure. Increase your vitamin and antioxidant intake.

Chapter 4

THE IMPACT OF SEX ON CARDIAC ARREST
(Why Men Die On Top During Sex).

We must examine this topic since comprehending this perplexing occurrence and avoiding the risk factors are just as important as therapy. The sudden death of males during sexual intercourse has been a long-standing mystery for many centuries. Many things have been attributed to it as an immediate or distant cause. (s).

We live in an information age, and I believe it is past time for males to learn what goes wrong and how to avoid it. Understanding the neurological systems by which the body initiates erection and ejaculation would be quite beneficial in helping you comprehend how this heinous act happens.

Erection And Ejaculation Physiology

Without initially comprehending how the body manages the fascinating occurrence of Erection and Ejaculation, one may not be able to realize how unexpected death happens during sex.

Both erection and ejaculation must be successful for a guy to have sexual enjoyment. However, the biological system regulates these two actions in separate ways. The brain controls almost all of the events that occur in the body. The brain delivers signals to the target organ through the Nervous system, which is a wire-like network.
The nervous system is divided into two pathways: parasympathetic and sympathetic nervous systems. In the body, these channels nearly usually conduct conflicting activities. The parasympathetic nerves begin and sustain an erection during

reproduction. Ejaculation, on the other hand, is governed by the sympathetic nervous system, which also governs the motions of the heart and blood vessels. Several weird things happen during ejaculation.

With the discharge of sperm, the Sympathetic nerve induces the muscles of the sperm storage tank, epididymis, and Vas deferens to contract violently. However, since the same nerve controls the movements of the heart and blood arteries, it generates certain undesired consequences, including:

- A sudden increase in cardiac activity and, in rare cases, a brief halt of heart rhythm.
- Boost your heart rate and pulse rate.
- Blood vessel constriction causes an increase in blood pressure.
- Increase Sweating
- Exhaustion without warning

How Men Die Suddenly While Having Sex.

Sudden death happens as a result of a misreading of signals (electric impulses) that reach the heart as a result of the sympathetic nervous system acting on the heart and blood vessels. (Cardiac Arrest). This is more common in adults over the age of 40. As a consequence, unexpected death during sex is caused by **Cardiac Arrest.**

Factors Contributing to Sudden Death During Sex.

Sudden death during sexual intercourse is a cardiac condition that may be exacerbated by the following factors:

Sexual Greed

According to studies, almost 85% of men who died on top perished outside their houses, mostly in hotels, and the majority of them died on top of women who were never their spouses; primarily workplace secretaries, girlfriends, prostitutes, and so on. In a time-sensitive location such as a hotel, most men engage in unremitting sexual activity to meet up or have enough turnover for the night. Sexual avarice stimulates the use of sex-stimulating medicines, which do not protect the heart. The heart stops while attempting to ejaculate by whatever means possible.

Sex-Stimulating Drug Use

Sex-evoking medicines, such as Viagra, all have the same mechanism of action. They promote erections by boosting nitric oxide levels, which is a potent vasodilator. This action causes the medications to increase penile blood flow and consequently erection. They also assist to alleviate the symptoms of sexual dysfunction, such as impotence, via this activity.

However, since they have no impact on the Sympathetic nervous system, which produces ejaculation, they do not protect against cardiac arrest. These medicines should ideally be provided after an individual's cardiac state has been assessed. A person with cardiac dysfunction, angina, coronary artery disease, or other associated heart issues may give up after attempting to ejaculate to alleviate the drug-induced penile erection. Sexual greed also contributes to this heinous consequence.

Disorders of the Metabolic or Cardiovascular System:

Cardiac issues and other chronic metabolic health concerns might increase the risk of cardiac arrest during sexual intercourse. For example, a man suffering from Angina Pectoris (a heart illness characterized by sudden intense sensations in the chest) may die abruptly from Myocardial Infarction, a complication of angina.

HOW TO AVOID SURPRISE DEATH DURING SEX

Understand Your Health Status:

Unfortunately, most individuals judge their medical health based on their outward appearance. True medical fitness goes well beyond that. As a result, detailed examinations and analysis by a doctor are required for you to have a solid understanding of your medical situation.

This is critical since one person's meal may be another person's death trap. Before prescribing most sex-related medications, persons must be properly assessed. Being conscious of your medical condition may help you avoid an unexpected death during sex.

Caution Should Be Exercised When Using Sex-Related Drugs

As previously stated, most sex-inducing medicines do not protect the heart. The medications were not intended to cause early frustration and death. Stop using drugs because a buddy or someone proposed it to you. Consult your doctor before introducing any foreign substance, medications or otherwise, into your body. If it costs money, spend it to learn about your health since ignorance will cost you more.

Spend Sex Time With Your Wife;

For the last 56 years, research in America has proven that men who stay with their marriages have healthier and longer lives than those who have an uncoordinated sexual routine. According to some of the studies, men are both emotionally and physically relaxed when having sex with their partners. There is also a strong feeling of accomplishment and eagerness to face the next day, which reduces the frequency with which sex-related medications are used.

Furthermore, since sexual enthusiasm may lead to diseases and unnecessary drug use, guys with a free lifestyle are more likely to have a sexual accident. According to research, impotence may make a guy emotionally unstable, putting his health in danger.

You Are the result of your friends.

Many guys now live in sorrow over the companions they had in the past. They wish such a period did not exist. They constantly want to change the past, but there is no way to do so. In their greatest regret, they imagined how it started, the companions who entered their life before the ravenous but sorrow-laden pleasure began. *You Are A Product Of The Friends You Keep, Friend.*

Stay away from your two friends who may still be delighted about discussing his sexual escapades after 40 years of life since a rat that swims with a lizard will remain wet long after the lizard is dried. Don't hang out with people who are self-certified physicians who can prescribe anything for you anytime you complain rather than recommending that you visit your doctor.

WHY DO MOST MEN DIE TOO EARLY?

Have you ever wondered why older men had longer sexual potency than males today? Isn't it concerning to you that elderly men had some of their children in their 70s and 80s when modern men are already frail at 60? Now here's a secret; a man's reproductive biology is controlled by hormones. Some hormones, such as **gonadotropins**, are generated in the brain, while the testis generates the major male hormone, **testosterone**. Testosterone stimulates spermatogenesis (sperm production) and other male sexual characteristics, such as the ability to maintain an erection.

Surprisingly, these hormones control one another. The gonadotropins in the brain encourage the testes to create testosterone, and when the latter reaches a particular level, it sends a signal to the brain to cease the former's production. If left alone, this feedback process will continue throughout life.

Unfortunately, most men ignorantly prioritize sexual pleasure above this fascinating gift of nature via the early usage of various sex-stimulating medicines and concoctions. Unbeknownst to them, several of these medications include the synthetic equivalent of the body's hormones. By injecting artificial hormones into the system, the same feedback process, i.e. inhibiting natural hormones in the body, remains active. If this behavior persists, it may take longer or possibly become difficult for the body system to restart regular production, even after the medicines are removed. In males, this might result in infertility or early sexual weakness.

Regrettably, the afflicted guys continue to take additional medicines, even mixtures, to undo the past out of ignorance, fear, and desperation. This is why, when it comes to your reproductive health, it is best to seek medical counsel.

Chapter 5

THE ROLE OF GOD AND DOCTORS IN DISEASE MANAGEMENT

There is an urgent need to simplify our understanding of God's role in illness care. I witnessed a strong difference of opinion about the role of God and physicians in sickness care. Some Christians and other religious organizations may make their members believe that going to the hospital is a sin or a sign of faithlessness in God's ability to cure them via beliefs and poorly understood teachings. Some people even see physicians as demons who must be shackled.

I had never been a victim until recently when a patient's experience opened my eyes to the devastation caused by such ignorance-induced fights. It was the case of a guy who had TB related to HIV-AIDS infection, based on clinical indicators and medical investigation results. Surprisingly, when the guy exited my examining room, he ran into his wife, who was not there when I informed him of his medical report. She inquired, "What did the doctor say was wrong with him?"

The guy informed her that the doctor had diagnosed him with tuberculosis. The lady immediately contradicted it, saying, "It is not your portion; did you receive it from him?" Back to the sender, that is, the doctor (myself), Holy Ghost fire devour (who?). Of course, the doctor! Just look at me and you'll see disaster; maybe you'll become HIV-positive by fire. To be honest, the episode taught me the importance of educating people about physicians' responsibilities when it comes to illness.

People often give testimony in church that depict physicians as Satanic agents. Some individuals beg for physicians to be bound and sent into hell. Please understand that physicians are regular individuals like you, differentiated only by the information they gained via formal study, not by enchantments. As a result, most physicians will only provide you with scientifically validated information. Please keep in mind that if a doctor claims you have diabetes or HIV, he did not put it there. He will break free if you restrain him since he is innocent. Whatever a doctor says is based on the clinical facts and symptoms at his disposal.

That is the main reason Jesus never talked against physicians throughout his whole earthly career. He sat with physicians at the age of 12, listening and questioning them (Luke 2: 46), since he was going to be the healer of all ailments. He had them as ministry pals, which is why the book of Colossians 4:14 refers to Luke as the beloved physician.

SHOULD CHRISTIANS SEEK MEDICAL HELP?

Fundamentally, the medical profession is a gift of the Holy Spirit, not merely a vocation. It is a vocation within the ministry of assistance. Doctors and pastors provide the most important service that moves God's heart because they save lives. Doctors have a position in church ministry, according to God. That is why, in Jeremiah 8:22, He laments, *"Is there no balm (medication) in Gilead, no physician there?" So, why hasn't my people's daughter's health improved?*

The above scripture verse not only reveals the medical profession as a divine gift but also as part of God's plan for the health of his people. Little surprise, Jesus declared definitely in three distinct parts of the Bible; *"Those who are whole do not need a physician, but those who are sick do."* (Luke 5:32). Medical knowledge provides a foundation that demonstrates God's irrefutable healing power. That is why pastors continue to recommend individuals to physicians to certify supernatural healing. It is therefore neither a sin for a sick person to seek medical assistance nor is it a sign of God's fidelity.

Whatever talent one has on earth, it is only in measure, which is why man's capabilities cannot help but confront challenges, if even impossibilities, on occasion. As a medical practitioner, I recognize the many success stories that science and technology have told in the field of illness management. On the other hand, certain instances are classified as incurable terminal illnesses with an extremely dismal prognosis. I have also observed and proved God's power in proving man's judgment incorrect. Based on this, I concluded that *where man's understanding stops, God starts.*

God's Role in Disease Management

God created and completed human engineering. The human system's mechanism is so complicated that many things remain unknown. This is why the term "idiopathic" (unknown cause) is associated with scientific bewilderment. God creates mankind, whereas physicians are the roadside mechanics of the human body. Most of the time, your car's components or engine will get so damaged that roadside technicians will tell you absolutely that there is nothing that can be done and that your only alternative is to purchase new (original) parts from the manufacturer.

This also applies to humans; occasionally an organ or tissue is destroyed, and physicians conclude that the sickness is incurable based on scientific evidence. Some physicians may even go out of their way to provide the patient's expected death date. That is the explanation given by the roadside technician, and since human parts are not sold on the market, such messages are invariably accompanied by a sense of pessimism.

Nonetheless, Jesus recognized such situations and said in Mark 10:27, "*Such conditions may be impossible with men, but not with God; for with God all things are possible.*" As a result, knowing where to place your trust is critical. *Doctors can treat illness, but only to a certain extent; but God Can Where Man Cannot* That is why he is known as the GREAT PHYSICIAN. You must take notice of this distinguishing feature since so many people have ignored it and sunk their health.

You are aware that God has a role in mending that ailment. The medical sign of a snake hanging on a stick or cross, which was adopted by the Great Fathers of the Medical Profession, was inspired by an episode in the desert in which God instructed Moses to get a blue snake and place it on a cross so that anybody who looked at it would be cured.

The medical profession's forefathers accepted that physicians deliver pills and injections, but God heals. They took a page out of the wilderness healing experience and told you where to search for ultimate recovery. The book of Chronicles described the early death of a king who died of a foot ulcer, perhaps cancer because he thought God too subordinate to intervene.

And Asa, in the thirty-ninth year of his reign, became ill on his feet to such an extent that he sought the doctors rather than the Lord.

And ASA died in the forty-first year of his reign.

Regardless of your religious or scientific background, always accept God's role in your body's recovery. Even though science maintains there is no God, no one knows the genesis of man or why the man seems helpless in death. Of course, the same God who is still unknown to them has the answers to human biology and life in general. He teaches both preventative and curative medicine.

Never forget that it is God's heartbeat for you to live for at least 70 years. It is His Will that ailments and diseases stay away from your domain. That is undeniably true. All men are liars, but God is truthful. Never leave your health to chance, for where doctors fail, the Great Physician succeeds. He is, indeed, the same yesterday, today, and forever. Simply acknowledging and serving him will result in the fulfillment of the miracle of longevity and sorrow-free aging in your life.

And you shall serve the Lord your God, and he will bless thy food and thy water: and I (the Lord) will remove disease from among you.

Friend! You are predisposed to live a long life. I have poured forth this unique wisdom from the depths of my heart for your absolute health and freedom; gain it, use it, and don't forget to invite me to your 80th Birthday Celebration, which MUST come!!! CHEERS